Always With Me

The Guide to
GRIEVING DEATH
through
INTEGRATIVE
MEDICINE

Always
With Me

MICHELLE A. SMITH

NEW YORK

LONDON • NASHVILLE • MELBOURNE • VANCOUVER

Always With Me

The Guide to Grieving Death Through Integrative Medicine

© 2020 Michelle A. Smith

Published in New York, New York, by Morgan James Publishing in partnership with Difference Press. Morgan James is a trademark of Morgan James, LLC.
www.MorganJamesPublishing.com

ISBN 9781642795721 paperback
ISBN 9781642795738 eBook
ISBN 9781642795745 audio
Library of Congress Control Number: 2019939278

Cover and Interior Design by:
Chris Treccani
www.3dogcreative.net

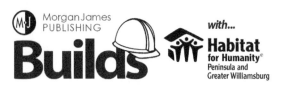

Morgan James is a proud partner of Habitat for Humanity Peninsula and Greater Williamsburg. Partners in building since 2006.

Get involved today! Visit
MorganJamesPublishing.com/giving-back

To my father,
who has always been with me.

TABLE OF CONTENTS

INTRODUCTION

It was Saturday, December 3, 2005. I was working and living in State College, Pennsylvania, and was excited for a weekend break. The previous week, my father had sustained a heart attack right before Thanksgiving, and my world had been rocked. How could my dad, at age fifty, have a heart attack? The Thanksgiving holiday was distorted from what it had always been, but we made the best of it nonetheless. Regardless, I was ready for the weekend. I was on my way out the door to the gym to get my Saturday started when I noticed a "one" flashing on the voicemail machine. I thought to myself, "That's strange." I almost walked out the door assuming it was for one of my roommates but, for whatever reason, walked over to the phone instead and listened to the message. I heard my grandfather's shaken voice on the message, "Um, hi, Shelly. It's Gramps. Your dad died last night. Please call home when you are able."

I was totally numb. How in the world could this possibly be? My dad was dead? I called home and talked to my uncontrollably sobbing mother. I hung up the phone. I walked out the door. I went to the gym. It took me hours to make that drive home that Saturday afternoon. It was the most surreal day of my entire life.

And so began my journey with the reality of death. Ever since that day, I've felt a strong calling to be present with people at the end of life and to help people manage the process of losing a loved one. It is a challenging but rewarding calling. Through the years, I've learned that there is no formula and there is no secret to navigating those rocky waters. However, I've also learned that at the center of the turbulence and in the middle of the crashing waves is a center, a home base that can be found. There is a still, small voice within that is always calling and leading us back to that center, back home.

For me, the way to find center, to find my way back home, has been through the modalities of integrative medicine. Amid the feelings of complete desperation, I attended my first yoga class almost a decade ago. I walked out of the studio feeling as if I had been wiped clean. I felt like someone had hit a reset button and I was, once again, operating from home base or a peaceful center within. That first yoga class led to me practicing yoga as a student for years before becoming a yoga teacher. Being a yoga teacher led me to obtain my Master of Science degree in yoga therapy. Working as a yoga therapist led me to pursue reiki training through the mastery level and to become certified as a vibrational sound therapist using the Tibetan singing bowls on the physical body to help people know internal happiness and peace. Each modality has taught me that all roads lead back to a center or home within that is total peace regardless of circumstances, sensations, judgments, or thoughts.

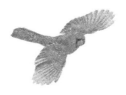

CHAPTER 1

Feeling Alone

The words "You have cancer" are words nobody ever wants to hear. Nancy woke up one morning and received this call from her doctor. The doctor tried to console her by saying, "But I believe we caught this at an early stage, and I really trust that everything is going to be OK." For Nancy, that didn't matter. She had just been told that she had cancer. She had so many questions surrounding this new diagnosis. "What will treatment be like?" "Am I going to live?" "If I die, what is going to happen to my husband?"

There were so many thoughts and questions swirling through her brain and so many emotions pumping through her body that she did not know what to do. As the doctor said, "I want to see you in my office tomorrow to discuss next steps," Nancy thought to herself, "Oh my God. I have cancer."

The next day, Nancy arrived at her doctor's appointment. Nancy's physician showed her the results of her mammogram and told her, "Since we caught this at an early stage, you will likely only need surgery and radiation." Chemotherapy would likely not be necessary. However, the doctor shared, "But we will not know for sure until we go in and do the surgery." The uncertainty of not knowing was too much to bear. Nancy felt overwhelmed but so thankful that her husband was able to reassure her and say, "I am here with you, and everything is going to be OK."

Three weeks later, Nancy and her husband arrived at the hospital for her mastectomy. For Nancy, it was terrifying and humiliating to think about one of her breasts being removed. "What will I look like?" "Will my husband still think I am beautiful?" "Will my husband still love me?" As they were preparing her for surgery, Nancy's husband received a phone call from his doctor. "You have colon cancer." Nancy and her husband looked into each other's eyes as if to say, without any words needed, "What is going on? What did we do to deserve this?" They had to set all those thoughts and emotions aside as they began to wheel Nancy down the hallway for her surgery. Both Nancy and her husband felt so overwhelmed. They thought to themselves, "How are we ever going to get through this horrible situation?"

Nancy woke up from surgery and there in her room was her husband of thirty-eight years. For Nancy, he was her rock, her foundation, her everything. It took her a few minutes to realize where she was and then the flood of thoughts and emotions started swirling again. It was as if she was waking up into a horrible nightmare. Nancy just wanted to go back to sleep.

The days ahead after Nancy's surgery were tough. Dealing with the physical pain and the emotional pain of losing a breast were challenging. Worrying about her husband's diagnosis threw the whirlwind of thoughts and emotions over the top. But her husband reassured her, telling Nancy that "everything will be totally OK."

They had about a month to prepare for her husband's colon surgery. The plan, according to the colorectal surgeon, would be to remove the section of the colon that had cancer and then do a resection. If everything went according to plan, a colostomy would not be necessary. If things did not go according to plan, a colostomy might be required. Again, living with the uncertainty of the outcome was really challenging. But Nancy's husband was confident that everything would be totally OK.

The morning arrived for her husband's

surgery. Nancy was with him as he had been there for her. He went into surgery and came out with no colostomy. Hooray! However, as the days went by after his surgery, things appeared to be getting worse. Within a week, her husband had died. The surgeon told Nancy that his death was "due to complications from the surgery."

The gravity of everything that happened to her husband and Nancy within a two-month period was insane. Her husband's death put Nancy's breast cancer treatment into perspective and it no longer even registered to Nancy that she had cancer. For Nancy, her husband – her rock, her foundation, her everything for thirty-eight years – was gone. She felt so incredibly alone. Her husband was gone. She had cancer. Her status in society went from married to single literally overnight. Her married friends didn't know what to say to a newly single woman. A lot of people didn't want to talk to her because she had cancer and looking at Nancy was forcing them to confront their own mortality. Nancy wanted to die.

Nancy planned out her suicide. The plan brought her great peace. She was going to drown herself in a nearby lake because the thought of drowning seemed like the most attractive option. One day in a fit of anxiety, she decided to drown herself in a bathtub because she just wanted to get it done. Nancy got herself into the tub. She was ready to submerge herself under water when she heard a knock at the door. Nancy stopped. She got out of the tub. She threw on a robe and made her way to the door. It was Nancy's daughter, who said, "Something told me to come see you. Are you OK?" In that moment, Nancy knew that she was not alone. The thought that "something told her to come see me" gave Nancy enough hope to pull herself up by her bootstraps and get some help. She reached out to a psychologist at a local hospital. She started getting the help that she needed.

At the hospital, Nancy and her

psychologist began the process of unpacking everything that had happened to her over the previous months. Nancy was reassured that the thoughts and emotions she was experiencing were totally normal. Her psychologist also encouraged her to reach out to me, a yoga therapist in the health system who would be able work with Nancy using the tools of integrative medicine. Nancy thought to herself, "What is integrative medicine? How can yoga help me deal with the death of my husband and the incredible loneliness I am feeling?" Nancy was skeptical but after a few weeks decided to call me.

Nancy met with me at The House of Care, a home where cancer patients and their family members live while going through treatment. As soon as Nancy walked in the front door, she felt a tremendous peace. How in the world could a twenty-bedroom home filled with patients and families going through sickness and death have peace? Nancy was very intrigued.

I came out to introduce myself to Nancy, and we went into a room where I asked Nancy to share her story. Nancy told me about the ups and downs of the previous months of her diagnosis and her husband's death. I just listened. I created and held a peaceful space for Nancy to share her story. In that space, Nancy no longer felt alone. Nancy felt heard. She felt connected. She felt a sense of trust. In this connection, Nancy felt hope for the first time since her husband died. I acknowledged Nancy's pain and suffering yet offered a sense of hope that the tools I was going to share could help Nancy feel connected and loved. From that container of connection and love there was an opportunity for tremendous healing to take place.

Before Nancy left, I gave her a tour of the facility. Nancy was overwhelmed as we walked down the hallways and through the communal lounges and saw so many people going through treatment or dealing with the reality of disease and death. "I thought I was alone," Nancy said.

"Because of my situation managing this facility, it is easy to think everyone has cancer or is dying," I said. "Living and working in this space forced me to find internal peace at the age of thirty. I knew that if I did not figure out peace, I would not survive being in this space."

Nancy asked me, "How did you find internal peace in the midst of such a challenging environment?" And so began our journey together exploring how integrative medicine can help someone find peace in the midst of disease and death.

I introduced Nancy to physical postures, breathing exercises, and mindfulness practices to help her know peace during the incredible emotion surrounding her own cancer diagnosis and the death of her husband. Nancy fell in love with child's pose, a pose where you come onto your yoga mat, sink your hips back to your heels, extend your arms up straight, and walk your fingers to the top of your mat. Nancy loved how feeling her breath move into and out of her back created a grounding sensation and got her out of the stories swirling through her mind and into the present moment in her body. As emotions rose up, she was able to get into child's pose and feel a tremendous assurance and peace amid the thoughts and sensations swirling through her mind and body. In a very short time, Nancy was amazed at how the tools of yoga therapy could extend her a measure of peace during so many challenges.

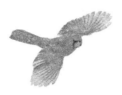

CHAPTER 2

My Story

I first came to know yoga from a place of desperation. At the age of thirty, I started working at a home for adult cancer patients going through outpatient chemo and radiation therapy. The job at that time and for the next seven years required that I live on site. Every day I was working and living with people whom I did not know. Some had surgery the next day. Some had treatable cancer. Some had no idea if they would live. Some had just found out they would be dead within six months. And most people had family members accompanying them who, in most cases, did not know how to handle the reality they had just been thrown into. Smoking in the building, drinking alcohol, exchanging narcotics, and domestic violence were a part of my world each week. Managing a host of personality disorders and other mental health conditions all under one roof where everyone was dealing with the stress and anxiety that accompanies disease was part of my job and life. It was insane. I knew that I needed to figure out internal peace as quickly as possible if there was any chance of me staying in the job. I wanted to stay. It felt like my calling.

My friend invited me to a yoga class. My initial thought was, "No, I need to be exercising more vigorously." However, after struggling with what I thought was a hamstring injury for several months, I decided to attend the class. At my first class, I had to modify the poses quite significantly, but I came away from the class not only feeling great physically but feeling as though I had been internally wiped clean and could enter back into my work and living space with a clean slate. I felt amazing. After that class, I dove headfirst into exploring yoga.

On weekends, I would travel to cities to practice in heated studios. My thought was, "If I can focus and breathe in a studio heated to 105 degrees with 40 percent humidity, I can focus and breathe anywhere." The heated practice became such a lifeline for me, allowing me to know peace in such a profound way that I would travel to Philadelphia on the weekends and sleep in my car just so I could practice both Saturday and Sunday. The practice helped me feel clean both mentally and in my physical body. The practice created a space between me and my surroundings that allowed me to be progressively less and less reactive and more and more free.

After practicing religiously as a student for four years, I embarked on my first yoga teacher training in 2013 to learn how to teach the practice that had become so instrumental to my own peace amid the craziness of work and life. The training was a wonderful experience that deepened my understanding of yoga. My practice became even more meaningful to me. It enhanced my ability to be with the uncertainty of disease and death and the deviant behavior that accompanies such stress. I fell so in love with yoga that I wanted to expand the opportunities to share it with other people. After hearing about a program at Maryland University of Integrative Health, I embarked on a Master of Science in yoga therapy to learn how to use the tools of yoga to meet the needs of individuals.

While I was completing my master's degree, the health system where I worked announced they would be starting an Integrative Medicine program. I reached out to the attending physician who was tasked with developing the program. We started working collaboratively to develop the program at a grassroots level. Slowly, physicians started referring patients to me to help them with a host of conditions: physical, mental, emotional, and spiritual. The opportunity to share the tools of yoga with patients was tremendous.

While working to help create the Integrative Medicine program, I had the opportunity to meet Jasmine, a chaplain in the hospital's Neonatal Intensive Care Unit who had started a Reiki program in the hospital. We started working collaboratively, including reiki under the umbrella of integrative medicine modalities. Seeing how well patients were responding to reiki, a hands-on healing energy practice, inspired me to learn how to share reiki with patients, and I embarked on both my Reiki 1 and 2 levels of training.

After completing my Reiki 2 training, things in my personal life started to deteriorate. In May 2017, I started to become very ill. I was hit with violent episodes of diarrhea and lost a significant amount of weight in a short period of time. One evening in June, I felt certain that I could feel a channel being burrowed between my rectum and my vagina. As that night progressed, I started to become very sick. I had a fever. My then fiancé and I were quite concerned. My fiancé drove me to the local Emergency Department at 3:30 in the morning to be evaluated for what I was sure was diarrhea coming out of my vagina. It was terrifying!

It took the entire day for doctors to tell me that the results of the CT scan were "inconclusive" but that there was a pocket of air by my rectum that needed to be evaluated. Shortly after, a young colorectal resident came into my cubicle in the Emergency Department and was able to lance and pack what turned out to be a perianal abscess. I was told to come back in three weeks to see the attending colorectal physician to be checked and that "there may be a fistula." I shared with them that I was certain there was a fistula because I had diarrhea coming out of my vagina, but because the fistula didn't show up on the CT scan, they gave me the impression that they did not believe what I was telling them. I was also told to follow up with my primary care physician (PCP) within three days.

Within three days, I was in my PCP's office trying to convince her that I in fact had diarrhea coming out of my vagina; however, because it didn't show up on the CT scan they were convinced that there was nothing wrong except some anxiety. They encouraged me to start taking Prozac. I tried Prozac, but the diarrhea still continued and the abscess was not fully healing. When I visited with the colorectal surgeon three weeks later, he said that he would need to see me back in three weeks to see if the abscess was fully healed. If not, there may be a fistula, but an MRI would need to be done to determine its presence.

Three more weeks passed, and the abscess was not fully healed. The colorectal surgeon set up the order for the MRI, and I had an appointment for the MRI scheduled within a week. I endured the MRI, and it was finally determined that I had a fistula that extended from my rectum to both my vagina and the perianal region of my body. The surgeon told me that the fistula was likely due to a "blocked anal gland" and not Crohn's disease because I "did not present like a typical Crohn's patient." He wanted to proceed with surgery to correct the fistula, but something inside me told me to wait. Thank God I listened.

In the meantime, I decided to do a better job with "preventative maintenance" and went to get my Pap test after years of being negligent. While on vacation in North Carolina, I received the dreaded call that my Pap had come back "abnormal due to HPV" and was told that "we will not know anything else until the biopsy is completed." I concluded immediately that I had metastatic cervical cancer due to all the symptoms that I had been experiencing and suffered intensely from overwhelming anxiety, becoming completely paralyzed with moving forward toward any medical resolve.

I mustered up the bravery to go for my biopsy, which came back with a high enough grade of abnormality that it necessitated a Loop Electrical Excision Procedure (LEEP). In this procedure, they use a hot wire to remove a portion of the cervix. The removed tissue is biopsied to determine if clear margins are obtained. On New Year's Eve weekend of 2017, I had the LEEP done and found out that clear margins were obtained and all the cancerous cells on my cervix were fully removed and no additional treatment would be needed. It was a tremendous relief.

Several weeks later, I had my colonoscopy, which finally brought medical resolve to the GI and fistula issues I had been having. As the attending physician walked in after the procedure, his look and words said everything. "Have you heard of the Crohn's & Colitis Foundation?" And so my journey with Crohn's began. Within a week, I was injecting myself with an immunosuppressant and taking an oral chemo and an antibiotic.

After receiving this diagnosis, my life started to make sense. Ten years earlier, I had a similar physical event, although with fewer complications. Three years after the death of my father in 2008, I started to get very sick with extreme diarrhea. After months of diarrhea, losing almost fifty pounds, my lower extremities swelling, and a third of my hair falling out, I started to heal. At the time, I did not receive a Crohn's disease diagnosis, but the diagnosis a decade later helped make sense of that event.

My father died very suddenly at the age of fifty from a massive heart attack. In the middle of the night, he got up to go to the bathroom and died on the toilet. My mother found him dead on the bathroom floor the next morning. The fact that my father's death was sudden and I lived a couple hours away allowed me to move through life for several years in denial of his death. Then in 2008, when I moved back to my childhood home for several months, I was forced to face the death of my father. The years of suppressed emotions arose in the form of what I now know was a Crohn's flare. At that time, I did not have the tools of integrative medicine to help me manage all the emotion.

The same week that I had complete medical resolve with the Crohn's diagnosis and complete healing from the LEEP procedure, I noticed my fiancé being very secretive with his phone. This was a huge red flag for me considering our history. Over a year prior, as we were buying our home and getting engaged, my fiancé came to me from what seemed like a place of brokenness to divulge that, as a pharmacist, he had relapsed into drug addiction. I was a mess and became an even bigger mess when I found out that there was infidelity involved with the relapse. Going against my inner voice, I continued in the relationship, trusting the words that my fiancé shared with me: "I am sorry, and I know I can do better." It was six months after this that I started getting sick, and looking back, I know that the way I managed, or didn't manage, the stress from the relapse and infidelity and the fear surrounding possibly losing my relationship with my fiancé was the trigger for my Crohn's flare.

So, after seeing the secrecy with the phone, I said to my fiancé, "I want to see your phone." Sadly, I could tell from the conversations he was having with a co-worker that the infidelity – this time with a new woman – was back. For months, I just lived with the weight of the infidelity, but when we met with Jasmine, the woman who was going to perform our wedding, my fiancé shared with me, "You will only ever be good enough ninety percent of the time, and I will always have to look for validation from other women." I spent several weeks pondering how to proceed. I understood all the complications of unraveling a wedding and splitting a home and all our possessions, and this made the decision challenging. However, I decided to end the engagement.

My yoga and reiki practices sustained me through two months of living with the man I thought I was going to marry knowing that the relationship we shared was dead. Amid the chaos of unraveling a shared home and wedding and processing all the emotions of losing the relationship that I had put hope and trust in, the practices of yoga and reiki gave me tremendous inner peace. I felt as if I was able to float through. Underneath everything was a great foundation of happiness, joy, and peace. I found that the modalities of integrative medicine that I used to help so many patients manage the emotions of disease and death were incredibly helpful in managing the emotions surrounding my own significant loss.

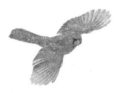

CHAPTER 3

Integrative Medicine Overview

Tammy was diagnosed with metastatic breast cancer at thirty-eight years of age. She had three boys and a loving husband and she was finally able to go back to college to finish her nursing program to become a registered nurse (RN). Life had been moving along so nicely and then the dreaded cancer diagnosis came along and seemed to turn Tammy's and her family's lives upside down.

Tammy navigated her mastectomy,

radiation, and chemotherapy with relative ease and was able to continue in her nursing program, graduate with honors, and achieve her nursing degree. She got a job at a local hospital as a cardiac care nurse. She and her husband built a beautiful house in the woods, and her boys were doing well in school and life. Things were good again.

Then, about three years after her initial diagnosis, Tammy started to feel a general dis-ease throughout her body. She quickly made an appointment with her doctor, and after some tests, it was determined that her cancer was back and in her liver. Tammy and her family were devastated by this news. The outcome of this recurrence was not good. The oncologist assigned to Tammy's care told her that she had approximately six months to live.

During those last six months of her life, Tammy and her family sought out alternative forms of medicine, not to necessarily eradicate her cancer, but to provide comfort to their souls and to feel some measure of peace. For

Tammy, modalities like yoga therapy taught her how to breathe through the tough days and find energy from postures when she was feeling low.

Tammy's husband, knowing that his wife was soon going to die, began to receive reiki sessions with a local practitioner. He described an incredible feeling of energy and peace during his reiki sessions and said that the sessions offered up a foundation that he knew would sustain him through his wife's death.

Within eight months, Tammy had died, but she radiated tremendous light and love up to her last moments on earth; while she was still able to talk, she expressed tremendous gratitude for all the peace and assurance she felt from yoga. Tammy's husband continued to receive reiki after Tammy died and often shared that the energy he received from the sessions sustained him during one of the most difficult events of his entire life. Through reiki, he was able to know peace and comfort during his wife's death. Through reiki, he shared that he felt a sense of connection to Tammy even though she was no longer in her physical body. He said that reiki helped open him up to new ways of seeing her presence in things of this earth.

I've been working at Geisinger Medical Center in Danville, Pennsylvania, to help create a new program called Integrative Medicine. The modalities that fall under the umbrella of integrative medicine include, but are not limited to, massage therapy, reiki, acupuncture, yoga therapy, and singing bowls. After years of working with these modalities, I believe the end goal of each is to help the receiver know internal peace. Each modality uses a different set of tools, but the end intention of each remains the same. The modalities that this book will focus on are yoga therapy, reiki, and singing bowls.

I spent two years studying to get my Master of Science degree in yoga therapy. The program, at Maryland University of

Integrative Health, was the first MS in yoga therapy on the planet. The tools of yoga therapy can be divided into three subsets: physical postures, breathing exercises, and mindfulness/meditation practices.

The physical postures are what most people think of when they consider yoga. In the West, this is what is most often promoted in the yoga world. If you look at the cover of yoga books or magazines, typically what is pictured are very fit people twisting their bodies into advanced postures. It is easy to look at these images and think that yoga is completely out of reach. The good news is that yoga is so much more than what you typically see on magazine covers or on the pages of social media.

Physical postures are also much broader than what most people see. Each posture can be stripped down to the basics by asking, "What is the intention of this pose?" Once you have the intention of the pose, it can be modified and done in almost any way, including in a chair. For example, a common pose in yoga is child's pose, which is a forward bending pose typically done on the floor with arms extended overhead, forehead pressed into the mat, and hips sinking back onto one's heels. This pose can be shifted to the chair and a table. A person can fold forward in the chair, place one's forehead on the table and simulate a similar stretch for the back side of the body. Having people in this pose breathe into the back is just one of many tools used for grounding, or to energetically come down from something like anxiety.

A patient or client coming to see me for the first visit will undergo an assessment of his physical body to determine, looking at his posture, where he is tight or weak, holding tension, under engaged, and so on. I look at his standing posture and his posture in selected poses for physical analysis. From that assessment, I choose physical poses to help meet the specific needs of the physical body.

Some of the common physical poses

that I use as tools with clients and patients are child's pose, standing forward fold, one-legged forward fold, and seated forward fold. All these folds, being face down, are used for grounding. Additionally, I use reclined bound angle, fish pose, and *savasana* for opening the front side of the body or poses to help give and receive energy. It is also important to not just work the spine in one plane with forward and backward folding. So, it is important to do spinal twist poses, such as seated spinal twist, reclined spinal twist, or triangle pose. Side bending poses such as side-bending child's and standing half-moon stretch the sides of the body and complete things by working the spine in all directions.

Additionally, I teach mudras, or hand gestures. Putting the hand in certain configurations has been shown to have an energetic effect on the bodily system. For example, sticking up the middle finger is a Western mudra. Go ahead and do it. What energy do you notice within you and around you? Bringing the tip of the thumb to connect with the tip of the ring finger has been shown to be very helpful for anxiety. Palms up is helpful for giving and receiving energy. Palms down is helpful for grounding and managing anxiety. A simple smile on the face is also shown to have an energetic effect on the person and the surrounding environment. Go ahead. Try it!

There are many breathing practices that are used in yoga therapy to help with a host of client and patient issues. Breathing practices are powerful because the breath interfaces directly with the nervous system. For example, if you hold your breath, chest breathe, or your breath is rapid and shallow, the sympathetic nervous system is upregulated. This is the part of your nervous system that triggers the stress response. If you belly breathe, extend your exhale, or breathe fully and evenly, the parasympathetic nervous system is upregulated. This is the part of the nervous system that helps you rest, relax, restore, and digest. Through different breathing practices, one can shift from sympathetic activation to parasympathetic activation.

When starting yoga therapy on a client, I perform a breathing assessment. If able, the client lies on the floor and is asked to assume his normal breathing pattern. The client or patient is observed. If the client or patient breathes into the chest or belly, that is noted. If the breath is short, shallow, rapid, long, deep, or even, that too is identified and noted.

Troubled or anxious clients are given breathing practices that help upregulate parasympathetic activation. One example of this is extended exhale through the mouth. It may be helpful for the patient or client to visualize breathing out of the mouth through a straw. Positioning the client or patient in a forward fold like child's pose and having him breathe into the back is excellent for grounding and managing anxiety.

When working with a practitioner, depressed patients or patients experiencing low energy may be given breathing exercises to help increase energy and joy. Breath of joy is a breathing practice where the person physically moves with the inhales and exhales, which has been shown to increase joy and energy in the system. *Kapalbhati* breathing is a breathing practice where one breathes in and out through the nose in conjunction with a rapid contraction of the abdominal muscles to help expel air from the lungs. Sitting and breathing with the palms face up is also effective for increasing energy and possibly helping manage depression. When dealing with the reality of death and loss, it is so easy to experience depression and the low energy associated with it. These exercises can be especially helpful for overcoming depression or managing the symptoms associated with it.

Mindfulness practices are very effective for helping the client or patient enter into a meditative state. The idea is that if you concentrate on something, thoughts and sensations that may ordinarily be a source of distraction cease, and one is able to enter into a state of complete union between mind and body through the breath where complete bliss is possible. The rise and fall of emotion associated with the comings and goings of thoughts and sensations settle, and everything just is. There is no division; there is no difference; there is only peace.

The type of mindfulness practice selected is based on what resonates most powerfully with the client or patient. If the person is highly visual, then a visualization mindfulness exercise will be selected. For example, the person could be systematically led through a guided visualization to a place that they associate with peace like the mountains or beach. If the person is highly auditory, then they will be given a practice such as listening to the sound of the breath, staying connected to that sound, and as thoughts and sensations creep in, shift awareness back to the sound of the breath. If the person is highly kinesthetic, then the mindfulness practice will be based on movement in the physical body such as a walking meditation or feeling the breath move into and out of a particular space in the physical body.

Reiki is a hands-on healing energy practice that has a relaxing or parasympathetic upregulating effect on the client or patient. In the Usai lineage in which I was trained through levels 1 and 2 and now into my mastery, we learn where to place the hands on the physical body to have a relaxing effect on the person receiving the treatment. Reiki is a very simple and pure form of energy work. Other than hands, no additional props or tools are needed to perform reiki.

Most patients who receive reiki fall asleep within minutes of the practice beginning, even if they are sitting in a straight back chair. Other clients or patients will describe the experience as if they are floating. Some mention at the end that they did not notice that my hands were no longer touching their physical body, as if their understanding of energy fields surrounding the body has been heightened.

The singing bowls are also part of integrative medicine. The singing bowls are done therapeutically under the umbrella of integrative medicine, which means they are placed on the physical body and struck with a mallet. The material used for the singing bowl along with the size, shape, and intensity the bowl is struck dictate the vibrations and frequencies that are created. The vibrations and frequencies have an energetic or shifting effect on the client or patient. Most clients or patients express improvements as better sleep and being able to manage stress, anxiety, and physical pain.

Each modality and the various tools of each modality resonate differently with different people. I find it most advantageous to expose the person to the entire spectrum of modalities and tools and then notice which ones have the most favorable effects for helping with the various issues and for helping the patient know a sense of internal peace.

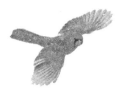

CHAPTER 4

What Is Yoga?

Talk therapy, such as cognitive behavioral therapy, has an important place in medicine, and I've found it to be amazingly helpful as I've navigated challenging times in life. The role of such therapies is to help a person process the storyline of what he is dealing with in life. Talk therapy works with the patient "inside the story." The modalities of integrative medicine, such as yoga therapy, have the potential to help the patient get "beyond" or "jump over" the story. There is a time and place for both.

Processing through the details of what happened in a situation is critically important, and this is a large part of talk therapy. For example, talking about the death of a loved one is a great way to verbally release emotion surrounding the death. Identifying potential "triggers" is also critical for working through challenging times.

The modalities of integrative medicine, however, help the patient in another way. Through the various tools that each modality presents, the person has the opportunity to tap into an internal space of bliss and peace that is beyond the physical, the mental, and the emotional. In yoga therapy, the various tools such as physical postures, breathing practices, and mindfulness exercises equip the person with things to focus on. Through that concentration, the waves of thoughts and sensations cease and the person may enter a meditative state.

In yoga therapy, each person has layers or bodies or sheaths that make up the person in entirety. The *annamayakosha* is the term given to identify the physical body. The *pranamayakosha* is the energy or breath body. The *manamayakosha* is the emotion body. The *vijnamayakosha* is the observer, and the *anandamayakosha* is the bliss body. The ultimate objective is to help the person move beyond the layers of physical, energy, mental, and emotional bodies to enter into a state of bliss and know that this state is accessible internally regardless of what is going on inside or outside. Knowing this yoga theory will help you better understand various experiences as you begin to practice yoga.

Hidden beneath the layers of physical and mental activity is a state of quiet awareness that is our true self. Peace, love, wisdom, and happiness can be found in this internal space. In the stillness of the inner self, we experience our connectedness to everything in the universe and to God. This blissful stillness is hidden inside every human being beyond the obvious. Few people experience it because they remain preoccupied with the objects, problems, and stories of everyday life. If we want to tap into this true self, we must learn, through the tools of yoga, how to quiet, control, and transcend the mundane preoccupations of the everyday world.

The union of the body and mind through the breath is yoga. Yoga is when the mind and body are in complete unison and the person is fully present in the moment at hand. There are no thoughts or bodily sensations that the person has reacted to pulling him out of the present moment. The true self is what remains when the noise and activity of the mind have been suspended or turned off. The waves of mental activity are like a curtain that hides the inner self. By calming and ultimately suspending these mental waves, we can uncover the true self. We learn to quiet these waves by concentrating on something "other," like the breath.

Yoga is the union of the individual self with the cosmic self or God. Through the practice of yoga, we have the opportunity to tap into complete connection with everyone and everything around us and, ultimately, with God. The ultimate goal of yoga is larger than simply to calm the mind – it is to connect the self with God. Since God is the center of all things, through the connection with God one is connected to all. This connection can be achieved through sustained and loving concentration on the thought of God. Arguably, all practices that calm and control the body and mind and help focus the attention on God are yoga.

Mary started working with me to use the tools of yoga therapy to help her better manage the anxiety and depression she was experiencing surrounding the death of her significant other who had died several years prior. Mary never fully dealt with all the emotion surrounding her partner's loss and consequently was struggling greatly from this significant loss in her life.

During her first session with me, I

placed Mary into reclined bound angle pose using props to make the posture restorative, meaning the props filled in the spaces between Mary and the floor, allowing her to fully surrender into the pose. This pose opens up her hips and chest, or heart, which are two places in the physical body where emotion is typically stored. I then had Mary place her hands gently over her heart. As soon as her hands were resting on her heart, Mary began to cry uncontrollably. The combination of the restorative pose with the powerful hand gesture allowed for emotion to well up. The props underneath her gave her the support she needed to feel these emotions, some for the first time.

After her session, Mary heard a still, small voice lead her to a gazebo on the hospital property, which had been erected in her significant other's memory after his death. He had been an employee in the health system where Mary was receiving her care. In that gazebo, Mary felt tremendously close to her deceased partner and was very grateful for hearing that still, small voice that led her to this space. This inner voice, sometimes called intuition, became louder after the release of her emotions and the silencing of her mind, which she learned to do through her yoga practice.

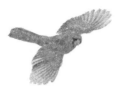

CHAPTER 5

Bend but Don't Break

When dealing with the death of a loved one, people often feel overwhelming sadness and sorrow and as if their lives have been unearthed. The physical postures of yoga therapy can be helpful in dealing with the feelings of loss. The symptoms the person presents with help determine which physical postures should be used to help manage the loss. This chapter will highlight many of the physical postures that I use for people dealing with the feelings of anxiety and depression that often accompany the loss of a loved one.

As discussed in chapter 3, mudras are hand gestures that have energetic effects on the being. There are many mudras that are helpful with feelings, such as depression and anxiety, associated with loss. The first one is *ksepana* mudra. Sit comfortably but be sure to keep your spine straight. The straighter the spine, the more sensitive you are to the energy moving through the body. Shift your attention to your breath and keep your palms facing upward to both give and receive energy. Then, after several breaths, put your palms together, interlock all fingers, but keep your index fingers straight and point the index fingers downward. Sit with your eyes closed for several breaths and simply notice the energetic effect on your being. Try to hold this for ten minutes. Continue to observe any shifts on your being as you stay grounded in your breath.

Some people notice immediate effects from mudras while others notice no effect at all as they start the practice. All the modalities of integrative medicine have an accumulating, or compounding, effect. Mudras are simple and can be incorporated into your life easily. Keep with the practice, be open, and notice any shifts that happen immediately or over time. Mudras are a powerful addition to your yoga practice and life.

Another mudra to practice is *uttarabodhi* mudra, for happiness and positivity. Put your hands together. Join the index fingers and thumbs and keep all the other fingers interlocked. Point the index finger toward the ceiling and the thumb toward the throat. After releasing the hands, place your hands on your thighs with palms face up. Take several deep breaths and take note of the effect the mudra had on your being. In addition to happiness and positivity, these mudras have the potential to shift one into a state of bliss or enlightenment and, in that state, obtain complete connection with the source of the universe.

Another mudra, for clarity of mind,

is *guyan* mudra. Make sure you are sitting comfortably with a straight spine. Bring the tip of the thumb to touch the tip of the pointer finger. Make sure all other fingers are straight. Turn the palms face up. Stay with this position for about ten minutes. When you are done, keep your eyes closed and hold your attention on the breath. You may notice that you feel lighter. You may feel more centered or grounded. But there is power in also just taking the time to simply notice how you feel.

Physical postures help counteract anxiety-driven depression, which is when anxiety is upregulating the sympathetic nervous system, causing energy to be expended and thus bringing you "down" or making you feel "low." Some postures help upregulate the parasympathetic nervous system, which helps you relax. Once this relaxation response kicks in, many people feel that instead of trying to escape their feelings, they can stay with them, which is essential to identifying triggers to their anxiety and depression. The path to getting to this relaxed place varies from person to person.

If you are feeling anxious or agitated, you might initially think that the best physical posture practice is one filled with relaxing, still, calming postures such as gentle forward folds. However, if your mind and energy are out of control, being still may be unmanageable and may end up making you feel worse. In these instances, I suggest starting your practice with dynamic postures such as sun salutations, warrior II, or a handstand. Downward facing dog is another great option for dynamic movement. Backbends and supported backbends are also great for anxiety and depression as they open up the heart and often the hip areas. Supported reclined bound angle is an example of a supported backbend that opens up areas of the body where emotions are stored and that has been shown to be helpful for both stress and anxiety. While in each pose, breath awareness is key. Deepening the inhalation is particularly helpful if you are struggling with depression or general sadness from the grieving process, as it stimulates and provides energy. Lengthening the exhale is especially helpful if you are dealing with anxiety because it upregulates the parasympathetic nervous system, which will help you calm, rest, and restore. The best way to learn about these postures is to visit a local studio, work with a yoga therapist one-on-one, or do some research online or through DVDs. Working with a trained yoga therapist like myself has huge benefits. Yoga therapists meet with you to assess and learn your specific needs and then create a plan of care using the tools of yoga.

As strange as it might seem to tell you to smile while grieving a significant other's death, try to smile just once in the privacy of your own space. Every position any part of our body assumes has an energetic effect on our being. If you wear a smile, your spirits lift the spirits of everyone around you as well. Try it. First, try it alone. Sit in a room alone with a neutral expression, and take a moment to just notice how you feel in this moment. Then, smile and take a moment to notice how you feel. Do you notice any shift? The shift may be subtle, but do you sense an energetic effect on your being after putting on a smile?

Next, wear a smile out and about. Notice how you feel as you smile at other people. Notice how other people respond to you when you smile at them. I think when you smile at another person, you establish an immediate connection, which has an invaluable effect in the soul. So, just try it.

Linda came to work with me after she lost her husband in a violent car accident. His death happened in the blink of an eye, and the reality of everything took months to sink in. Linda exclaimed, "My husband is dead" after weeks of working with me. She was finally processing the reality of his death after weeks of learning how to relax through the physical postures and breath work of the yoga practice. After some time, I suggested to Linda that she go into her bathroom, look at herself in the mirror, and smile. At first Linda thought the exercise seemed silly. However, one day it felt right to try to smile, and it was amazing how she felt. Linda noticed that the simple act of smiling made her feel a bit lighter and happier. The smile seemed to shift her disposition into a better place.

Once you feel more balanced, poses such as legs-up-the-wall and *savasana* can offer some much-needed rest. Keeping your eyes open or closed is dependent on the individual. If closing the eyes heightens vulnerability and increases anxiousness, then keeping the eyes open is a totally acceptable option.

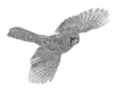

CHAPTER 6

The Power of the Breath

The breath interfaces with the nervous system in a profound way. You can use the breath to affect the nervous system and therefore affect your life. Take a few moments and sit in a comfortable seat with your eyes closed and turn your full attention to your breath. What do you notice? Are you holding your breath? Is your breath short and shallow or long and full? Where does your body expand as you inhale? Where does your body relax as you exhale? Do you reverse breathe? In other words, does your torso expand as you exhale and deflate as you inhale? What are all the qualities you can identify about your breath?

There are two parts to the autonomic nervous system that the breath directly affects. The sympathetic nervous system is the "stress response" or the "fight or flight response." This is the part of the nervous system that is necessary to help us flee from immediate danger. The parasympathetic nervous system is the part of the nervous system that helps us rest, relax, digest, and restore. Both parts are essential to our life and well-being. However, too often people live life in sympathetic overdrive. This means they are often in a state of heightened stress, and stress becomes the new normal. Breath awareness and regulation can help you shift from sympathetic overdrive to parasympathetic activation.

It is normal when dealing with the death of a significant other to be in sympathetic overdrive. The truth is you are processing a stressful and seemingly dangerous situation. There are so many scary questions that come up such as "How will I survive alone?" "Will I be able to pay for everything on my own?" "Will I be alone for the rest of my life?" The objective is to learn how to manage all that stress and upregulate the parasympathetic nervous system in the midst of the loss and perceived danger.

There are three parts of the torso that the breath moves into and out of. Three-part breathing is a great exercise for becoming aware of the three spaces that the breath moves into and out of. Lie on your back and bring both of your hands to your belly. As you inhale, feel your belly expand. As you exhale, feel your belly deflate. Next, bring both of your hands up to your rib cage. As you inhale, feel your rib cage expand. As you exhale, feel your rib cage deflate. Next, bring both of your hands to your upper chest or the space just below your collar bones. As you inhale, feel this space expand. As you exhale, feel this space deflate. Finally, lie with your arms alongside your torso and feel all three parts expanding as you inhale and deflating as you exhale. Practice this several times. Is there a space that you do not feel the breath moving into and out of?

Belly breathing upregulates the parasympathetic nervous system. Bring both of your hands to your belly. As you inhale, feel your belly expand. As you exhale, feel your belly deflate. Practice this for seven rounds. At the end of the seventh round, sit and simply observe how you feel. Chest breathing upregulates the sympathetic nervous system. If you identify yourself as a chest breather, practice seven rounds of three part breathing and see if, over time, you are able to shift your breathing from your chest area to incorporate your entire torso, especially your belly.

Extending your exhale upregulates your parasympathetic nervous system. Sit comfortably with your eyes open or closed and take a moment to count the length of your normal exhale. Once you have established that number, can you lengthen your exhale by one count? Then two counts? As you progressively lengthen your exhale, how do you feel? What do you notice about your state of being? Do you notice any softening in your physical body? Do you notice any ease in your thoughts and in your mind?

There are many other breathing practices that affect your overall being. Alternate nostril breathing helps to balance the right and left hemispheres of the brain and provide overall balance, stability, and peace to the entire system. If you are feeling unbalanced or in a state of dis-ease, this can be a very helpful breathing practice. Find a comfortable seat. Sit with your eyes open or closed depending on what feels more comfortable to you. Use your right hand and bring your thumb to your right nostril, your index and middle fingers to the space between your eyebrows, and your ring finger to your left nostril. Close off your right nostril and exhale through your left nostril. Breathe in through your left nostril, close off your left nostril, release your right nostril, and breathe out through your right nostril. Breathe in through your right nostril, close off your right nostril, release your left nostril, and exhale through your left nostril. This completes one round. Practice seven rounds and then sit and observe how you feel after the practice. Close your lips and breathe in and out through your nose. Breathe in through your nose deeper than normal. Exhale slowly through your nose while the muscles in the back of your throat are slightly constricted.

Kapalabhati breathing literally means skull-shining breath. Although the effects of this breathing practice vary from person to person, typically people feel a heightened sense of alertness and energy after the practice, making this ideal for those times you are struggling with depression. *Kapalabhati* breathing consists of short, forceful exhales and slightly longer, passive inhales. The exhales are accompanied by contracting the abdominal muscles which helps to expel air out of the lungs. The inhale happens naturally. Bring your attention to your belly. Quickly contract your lower belly pushing air out of your lungs. Then release the contraction so the belly relaxes and air is returned into your lungs. Repeat this practice eight to ten times at first and slowly increase the number of rounds as you advance in the practice.

Lion's breath is a great practice for releasing heat from the body and mind. For example, if you are physically overheated, this is a great practice. If you are emotionally overheated (for example, from anger), this is also a great practice. For this exercise, find a comfortable seat. Breathe in fully through the nose, and then as you exhale open your mouth, stick out your tongue fully, and forcefully release the air through your mouth. Repeat this for seven rounds, and take a few moments to notice how you feel.

Jim worked with me for over a year only using breathing exercises because he was paralyzed. His wife died in the car accident that left him paralyzed. When he first started working with me, he was very depressed about the reality of his situation. At fifty years of age, he was confined to a wheelchair and living in a nursing home and his wife was dead.

One of the exercises I introduced to Jim was alternate nostril breathing. Jim was unable to lift his right hand up to his nose, but I believed that this practice would provide the concentration and balance needed to help Jim find peace in the midst of all the challenges he was facing. I had Jim visualize everything that his right hand was unable to do. Amazingly, Jim felt a profound sense of peace and bliss after practicing this exercise for several weeks. Jim was able to relax and in that space begin to safely deal with the emotions that came up surrounding his situation. Jim was on his way to healing the emotions and sensations stemming from his profound loss.

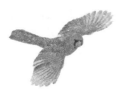

CHAPTER 7

Concentrate to Meditate

Mindfulness is the act of concentrating on something. That act of concentration has the potential to silence the waves of thought and sensation in the body and mind. Through that silencing, the opportunity opens to enter into a meditative or bliss state. There are many different types of mindfulness practices. Some practices will resonate with you more than others.

A body scan meditation is where your

attention is systematically guided to different parts of your body. Lie on your back, face up, and find a comfortable position. It may be helpful to place a pillow or bolster under your knees. For each location where you shift your attention, take one inhale and one exhale. To begin, bring your attention to the space between your eyebrows. Shift your attention to your throat. Bring your awareness to your heart. Shift your attention over to your right shoulder. Move your attention down to your right elbow. Now shift your attention down to your right wrist. Move your awareness to the middle of your right palm. Bring your attention up to your right wrist. Shift your attention up to your right elbow. Bring your attention up to your right shoulder. Shift back over to your heart. Now move your attention to your left shoulder. Move your attention down to your left elbow. Shift your awareness down to your left wrist. Bring your awareness down to the middle of your left palm. Shift your attention back up to your left wrist.

Shift up to your left elbow. Move up to your left shoulder. Bring your attention back over to your heart. Move your attention down to your belly button. Shift your attention down to your pelvic floor. Move your awareness over to your right hip. Shift down to your right knee. Move down to your right ankle. Bring your attention to the middle of your right foot. Move back up to your right ankle. Move up to your right knee. Shift up to your right hip. Move over to your pelvic floor. Shift your awareness over to your left hip. Move your attention down to your left knee. Bring your attention down to your left ankle. Move down to the middle of your left foot. Move up to your left ankle. Move up to your left knee. Bring your attention up to your left hip. Move your attention back over to your pelvic floor. Move up to your belly button. Bring your awareness up to your heart. Now back up to your throat. Now up to the space between your eyebrows. Lie comfortably for five breaths. With each inhale, feel your entire body expand. With each exhale, feel your entire body relax. How do you feel?

Some people connect deeply with sound and that helps facilitate a deep concentration and possibly an entry into a meditative state. Find a comfortable position, either on your back or sitting in your chair. Ideally, find a space with as little noise as possible so your full attention can be on the sound of your breath. You can either keep your eyes open or closed. Take an inhale and keep your awareness on the sound of your inhale. Take an exhale and keep your awareness on the sound of your exhale. Does the sound of your breath remind you of anything? Take seven breaths. Seven inhales. Seven exhales. If you find your attention being pulled away from the sound of your breath by a thought, sensation, or something in the room, practice bringing your full attention back to the sound of your breath. After completing the seven breaths, how do you feel?

Other people who are highly visual connect deeply with visualization mindfulness practices. One example that blends visualization with the breath is to identify a color that you want to associate with the breath. Lie on your back in a comfortable position or sit comfortably in a chair. You can keep your eyes open or closed. As you inhale, visualize the color associated with your breath moving up through your nostrils, down your throat, and into your lungs. As you exhale, visualize the color associated with your breath moving out of your lungs, up your throat, and out of your nose. Repeat this practice seven times. At the end of the seventh breath, take a moment to breathe normally and reflect on how you feel.

Some people prefer movement with their mindfulness practice, particularly if they find sitting still to be quite challenging. If you are struggling with high levels of anxiety, movement may be especially helpful when you start mindfulness work. A walking meditation may be a practice you connect with if stillness is a struggle. You can do this inside. If you are inside, I suggest removing your shoes so that your feet make a full connection with the floor beneath you. Begin walking around the room and count the number of steps you take with each inhale and the number of steps you take with each exhale. Can you increase the length of your inhale and exhale by at least one step? Repeat this exercise for five minutes. Then sit comfortably, assume your normal breathing, and take a few moments to notice how you feel.

You can also do the walking meditation outside. Either do the same practice prescribed for inside outside or try a different practice outside. As you are walking, find something that interests you. Now try to engage all your senses in the object you have identified. What do you see? What do you hear? Is there a sound associated with this object? Is this object appropriate for eating? What, if anything, do you smell? After engaging in this mindfulness practice, find a comfortable seat and reflect on how you feel.

I led a walking meditation for a group of widows and widowers around the hospital campus where I work. Sometimes it is very helpful to practice these exercises in the company of others to realize that you are not alone in your challenges and also to feel the energy of the group practice. Other people can also serve as wonderful sources of inspiration and motivate us on our path of healing.

After the experience, Sarah, one member of the group on the walking meditation, shared with the group her story and how the exercise was helpful. She shared that the exercise brought to her awareness of how much time she spends "in her head" pondering the loss of her husband and how many little things she misses around her that could bring her a profound sense of joy. She shared that she noticed a leaf on the sidewalk in the shape of a heart and in that moment felt her husband's presence with her. She said, "Before this walking meditation I would have likely missed the leaf because I would be in my head feeling sorry for myself about so much." She shared that she realizes she has likely missed many moments of joy and his presence with her because she was not able to notice them.

Concentration, like the practices outlined here, can be the portal into a meditative state. In a meditative or bliss state, there is a complete wholeness. There is a total connection to everyone and everything around you. There is a feeling of complete love, joy, and peace. There is a total unity with all things past, present, and future. There is no concept of time. There is an absence of space or separation. You are residing in another dimension that is infinite and eternal. You will know this space by experience. You will just know.

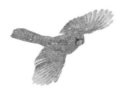

CHAPTER 8

Hands-On
Healing Energy

Reiki is a "hands-on" healing energy practice that is a transfer of healing energy from one person to another from the Divine or force greater than oneself. The person offering reiki is literally a channel through which the healing energy flows. Both the provider and receiver, if sensitive to it, will feel energy moving. Some people describe the sensation as "expansive" or as if they are bigger than what they previously understood their physical bodies to be. Many people comment that when the hands are removed it still feels as if the hands are on the body. People comment that their understanding of where their physical body ends changes, and they feel "bigger than" themselves.

All of the modalities of integrative medicine have the same intention, helping a person experience being bigger than himself. The intention is to help the person come into a space where he is bigger than a thought and bigger than a physical sensation. In this space, the person is experiencing the eternal. The person is in a dimension that is outside space and time and is infinite. It is this space that we all have in common. It is in this space that we all ultimately reside.

I have the amazing privilege to work with patients throughout Geisinger Medical Center. I have witnessed some amazing moments of connection when offering reiki to patients. One day I was working with patients in the outpatient chemotherapy infusion suite. I walk around the infusion suite asking patients if they are interested in receiving reiki as a means to help relax in what can be a charged environment. Many patients accept. This particular day, there was a man, alone, sitting in his infusion chair. When I asked if he wanted reiki and explained exactly what it is, he accepted immediately. The way we practice reiki in this setting is for five minutes my hands are placed on the top of the head and for five minutes my hands are placed on the shoulders. As soon as I placed my hands on the top of his head, he reached his hands up to touch mine. He started crying. I asked him if he was OK. He said, "These are tears of joy. I usually feel so alone, and I feel such a connection." I asked him to elaborate. He shared, "I feel a strong connection to you, and I also sense my deceased mother's presence right now." It was an amazing moment to share with this human being. As I walked away, we smiled at each other a smile of knowing that something miraculous had just taken place.

I work with patients who are admitted to the hospital. There was a man who was admitted to the inpatient palliative medicine/hospice unit who had nobody present in his life. His family and friends had all abandoned him. I was called by Care Management to reach out to this patient and use the integrative medicine modalities to help him feel loved and connected. On my first visit, I offered him both a singing bowl session and reiki. I was not sure if one or both would resonate with him. I did a thirty-minute singing bowl session and then ten minutes of reiki. As soon as I placed my hands on top of his head, he reached up with his hands to touch mine and tears started to stream down his face. He whispered to me, "I feel love."

Reiki is very powerful when navigating through the reality of the loss of a loved one. On a practical level, physical touch from another human being, assuming that physical touch is not a trigger, can feel very helpful when dealing with loss. Just take a moment to reflect on how nice a hug feels when you are dealing with something challenging. It is a physical reminder that you are not alone. Realizing that you are not alone can be very helpful in processing the emotions of grief. It creates a sense of safety and security for those emotions to come up, be processed, and move through you.

Additionally, reiki does allow for a moving of good, healing energy through the provider to the person receiving. Many people report a sensation of "floating" in this good energy space. Being in the space of good energy allows the person receiving reiki to identify with something other than the emotions surrounding grief, if for only a few moments. It allows the person receiving reiki to know that there is something else they can identify with and drop into for those emotions surrounding grief to be processed. There is a connection to something much greater than oneself. In this healing space of connection and bliss, one is potentially more open to seeing the presence of a loved one in his life.

Lastly, it is reasonable both financially and time-wise to get certified in reiki. Through the certification, one learns how to practice self-reiki so that it can be done without being dependent on a provider. Additionally, the act of giving reiki to another person is very healing as well. As the provider you can feel the healing energy pass through you. It is also always helpful to serve others to get your mind off yourself.

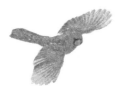

CHAPTER 9

Good Vibrations

Therapeutic singing bowls are bowls designed specifically for vibrational sound therapy and differ in many aspects from traditional Tibetan bowls. The idea behind crafting a refined instrument for both pure tone and strong vibration came after working with thousands of traditional bowls, some designed for eating, storage, and many other purposes. These sometimes very primitive singing bowls of antiquity are truly unique from bowl to bowl. A more precise instrument was needed for a more effective treatment. Creating a bowl for a standardized system required both knowledge of traditional bowls as well as modern science and engineering.

Therapeutic singing bowls are one of a kind. They are the first "singing bowls" designed as a tool to provide application of vibration directly to the body. In therapeutic singing bowls, the metal mixture is modified to provide an extremely resonant alloy. The notable differences in tone between a therapeutic singing bowl crafted for vibrational sound and a modern Himalayan singing bowl are the subdued volume and the purity of tone. Therapeutic bowls will have a cleaner sound due to the finishing process while still having a rich multitude of overtones. The smoothing out of the bowl's surface removes some of the natural variances that define these overtones, allowing the dominant tone of the bowl to really stand out.

Vibrational sound therapy combines powerful vibration and tones to induce an immediate relaxed state. The induction of the sound waves directly into the body, along with soothing ambient tones, is such a strong treatment that clients report effects ranging from a meditative state to deep relaxation. By placing the "therapeutic" singing bowls directly on the body and using correct techniques, a practitioner engages with their client both physically and aurally. This is also known as vibrational sound massage.

Vibrational sound therapy has been shown to be effective for quickly introducing deep meditative states. It is also known for reducing depression and sleep issues. It helps with easing blockages and tension. It is great for reducing stress; heightening focus; gaining a clear mind; calming the mind, body, and spirit; and boosting creativity and connection.

One of the patients I work with received an hour-long vibrational sound therapy session. After the session, she came out into the lobby area with tears in her eyes. She exclaimed that when the bowls were close to her heart, she felt the presence of her husband. She shared that she felt close and connected to him during the vibrational sound session.

As is the case with the other modalities of integrative medicine, the therapeutic singing bowls upregulate the parasympathetic nervous system. Being able to find relaxation in the midst of grieving the loss of a loved one is so helpful for staying at peace and managing the wave of emotions and sensations that such an event unearth. Like the other modalities, the singing bowls have the potential to drop a person into an expanded, meditative, transcendental state of being. In that space, a person feels bigger than body and bigger than mind. That person is in a dimension bigger than the physical and bigger than the mental. In this space, connection to the true essence of all other beings is inevitable. This is so beneficial for someone dealing with the loss of a loved one because in this space seeing the presence of your loved one in your earthly life is totally possible as you are one with all things outside of time.

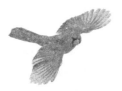

CHAPTER 10

The Process of Healing

Grieving the loss of someone you love is difficult. While there is no right or wrong way to grieve, there are healthy ways to cope with the pain and feel less alone. Not coping with the grief can lead to larger issues down the road if emotions are suppressed.

Give yourself time to accept what has happened. There is no schedule for when you should feel certain emotions over others. Choose to stand up for you and the rest of your life and choose to move on. You don't have to figure out how you're going to get through the rest of your life. Just focus on staying in the game and moving forward now. It is normal to cry and be depressed, but you need to keep putting one foot in front of the other.

After the initial shock of any type of trauma, there are, of course, the various stages of grief that everyone goes through, including denial, rationalization, anger, and acceptance. For those who are on this journey, it is important to have faith in yourself and the inner compass that guides you. If you do this, you'll understand that opportunities for growth and happiness lie in the most unexpected places, ready to be seized if you're open to recognizing and embracing them. I don't believe we ever get over a significant loss, but we do learn to move through it, live with it, and perhaps even use it creatively to find our life's purpose and harvest its lessons.

In healthcare and society in general,

our drive to save lives eclipses care around the dying process, and consequently, we are uncomfortable talking about death. In the same way, our focus on the health of the physical body trumps that of our mental well-being, and as a result mental health conditions are poorly understood and stigmatized. Putting all these things together helps explain why some people do not process or work through grief. But processing it all is incredibly important.

Through writing, through words, through movement, through tears, through screaming at the top of your lungs or whispering to the wind, it is significant to work through grief. The way into grief was very narrow, but the way through is up to you.

As an introvert myself, when I was mourning the death of my dad, so many of the traditional parts of the mourning process felt very invasive to me. For instance, people coming over to my house after the funeral felt overwhelming. I know that everyone meant well, but having people in my home, some of whom I barely knew, felt very unsettling. I suppressed many emotions surrounding my dad's death and lived in denial for several years. When the emotions arose inside of me three years after his death, I had what turned out to be the first significant Crohn's flare of my life.

I'm going to be as clear as I possibly can: you have permission to grieve. Grieving does not mean that you wallow in despair for the rest of your life. It means you give voice and you give space to the horrors you have endured and bear witness to them in whatever way that unfolds.

Physical movement in yoga can keep you healthy during a stressful time. Even though grief is primarily a psychological reaction to loss, your nervous system still responds as if the event was an attack on the body. For this reason, the modalities of integrative medicine that interface with your nervous system and help upregulate the parasympathetic component are very helpful to help the body rest, relax, digest, and restore through the grieving process.

You don't have to feel guilty about your grief. Special days, objects, and scents can bring up very difficult memories, and this should not create a feeling of shame. You are deeply missing your loved one, and you are emotionally fragile. Each time you apologize, you are basically sending yourself a message that you are doing something wrong. Continue to work through the process of grief and trust that, in time, new levels of freedom will emerge.

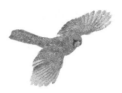

CHAPTER 11

Going Beyond and into Love

I gave Angel thirty consecutive days of reiki as part of my reiki mastery training. When I arrived the first night, I sat down on the couch, and Angel said, "I have something to tell you." Angel shared, "I so appreciate the timing of things. The last day of our thirty days of reiki is my husband's trial. He was caught driving with a suspended license and the county where this happened wants to make an example out of him and sentence him to prison for either thirty straight days or fifteen weekends."

Angel was terrified as she shared this news, scared both of being judged by me and of the reality that she faced. She shared, "I am scared to be alone." Even though Angel was not facing the physical death of her husband, she was facing the uncertainty of how things would unfold and the real potential of being separated from and losing the husband she always knew. I began the session by placing my hands over Angel's eyes and immediately Angel began to cry. As I placed my hands on different parts of Angel's body, I could feel energy pouring out of them. I sensed that Angel was very depleted from the months of worry and stress surrounding the uncertainty of the situation with her husband. The entire first session, I heard the words in my soul, "Everything is going to be OK."

Once the session was over and Angel sat up, we began discussing the session and everything that happened. Angel shared that she could feel the energy pouring into her body through my hands and she felt this assurance that everything was going to be OK. And thus began our thirty-day journey of progressively entering into the space of collective consciousness where all things are possible. If you think something, someone else knows what you are thinking. If you feel something, it is because it is real in the body or reality of the person in front of you. And you do not need to be in the physical presence of someone to have these mystical occurrences. You just need to have faith and believe that it is possible. You just need to have faith and believe that it is real. As the days progressed, Angel started feeling stronger. Angel articulated that she felt as though regardless of the outcome of the trial, she knew she would be OK. Physically, I could feel during the reiki sessions that Angel was less depleted. If I performed distance reiki, Angel could actually feel when I was visualizing my hands on that part of her body.

Angel shared more and more as well that as we were progressing through the thirty days of reiki, she felt close to her mom. She said on multiple occasions that her mom visited her in dreams. Angel also noticed more and more synchronicities in her life, which gave her tremendous assurance that if we are in the right place with ears to hear and eyes to see, we are privy to the beautiful connectedness of everything. We tap into the realm of collective consciousness where all beings, those in their physical bodies and those who have crossed over, are all one.

Reiki opened up Angel to this space of complete connection. It gave her tremendous assurance in waiting to know the outcome of the trial, knowing that even if her husband went to prison, she was never truly alone, and they would always be connected even if not in each other's physical presence. I was elated with the insight that Angel gained through the thirty days of reiki. As the days and weeks passed by, Angel more and more quickly surrendered into the reiki practice. Angel was able to express that surrendering into my hands during the reiki sessions was simply a picture of the ultimate surrendering into the space of collective consciousness, of universal energy, of God where we are all connected and we are never alone. Angel shared that she felt as though in this space, she was completely dissolved into a container of love. This realization is the goal of all the modalities of integrative medicine. This is the understanding that practitioners of integrative medicine hope their patients realize. Dropping into the space that Angel articulated is entering into the dimension of peace, love, and healing. It is the dimension where we are all one for eternity. It is a realm of total connection, joy, and bliss. It is the space that so many people whose stories were shared on the pages of this book came to know after practicing peace. It is a realm where they felt connection to those who have passed on and through the connection knew that they were never alone and always with everyone past, present, and future.

I was able to share my own experiences with Angel of feeling this connection. When my father died in 2005, on the night of his viewing I glanced over my shoulder and looked at one of the flower arrangements that seemed to stand out as significant. Woven into one of the arrangements was a cardinal and in that moment I just knew that this was significant and would be symbolic of my father's continued presence in my life even though he was no longer in his physical body. From that moment forward, a cardinal was present in various forms at every significant event and juncture in my life. At my brother's fortieth birthday party, there was a painting of a cardinal outside the room where the party was being held. One Father's Day when I was driving back from Virginia to Pennsylvania, I passed a fleet of five passenger buses and the bus line was "Cardinal." When my fiancé divulged in front of our wedding officiant that I would never be enough and he would always have to find validation from other women, there were cardinal napkins at the center of the table. Ever since my father's physical death, I have always seen and felt my father's presence. I have known, without any doubt, that a component of my father, and a component of all human beings, is eternal and always with us.

ACKNOWLEDGEMENTS

To the Morgan James Publishing team: Special thanks to David Hancock, CEO & Founder for believing in me and my message. To my Author Relations Manager, Gayle West, thanks for making the process seamless and easy. Many more thanks to everyone else, but especially Jim Howard, Bethany Marshall, and Nickcole Watkins.

THANK YOU!

Thank You for reading my book, *Always With Me: The Guide to Grieving Death Through Integrative Medicine.* This is not the end but possibly just the beginning of your healing journey. Wherever you are in this healing process, I would love the opportunity to further help you. Please email me at msmithsvhoh@gmail.com to schedule one free yoga therapy for grief session through online video conferencing.

ABOUT THE AUTHOR

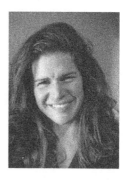

Michelle began a position as resident manager of a lodging facility for patients and families on a hospital campus in central Pennsylvania at the age of thirty. Feeling completely overwhelmed living and working in such a charged space, Michelle knew she needed to figure out internal peace. When Michelle suffered from a hamstring injury, a friend encouraged her to try yoga. Reluctantly, Michelle attended her first class thinking, "I am not flexible enough to do yoga." Her first teacher pointed out, "Well, that's kind of the point." After her first class, Michelle not only noticed the physical benefits of just doing modifications of some of the poses, but also felt as if she was "wiped clean" internally. She felt as if someone had hit a reboot button, and she was able to return to her work and living space from a much clearer and healthier space.

After practicing yoga as a student for two years, Michelle pursued her first teacher training at Melt Hot Yoga in Edwardsville, Pennsylvania. The benefits of yoga for herself and her students were so great that Michelle next completed her Master of Science in yoga therapy at Maryland University of Integrative Health. In her last few months of her master's program, the health system where Michelle worked announced that they would begin creating an Integrative Medicine program. Michelle reached out to the attending physician tasked with its creation, and they began collaborating to create what is today a fully operational Integrative Medicine program.

Michelle has completed additional yoga trainings, is pursuing her reiki mastery, and is a certified vibrational sound therapist. The modalities of yoga therapy, reiki, and singing bowls have had a profound effect on Michelle in terms of healing from the loss of her father and the loss of hundreds of patients who became friends and surrendered to death through the disease of cancer. Additionally, the modalities helped Michelle find peace as she was simultaneously dealing with her own cervical cancer scare, a Crohn's disease diagnosis, and a fiancé who relapsed into drug abuse and infidelity.

Michelle feels incredibly blessed to work with so many patients and families navigating through the extreme challenges of disease and death. Michelle shares, "Every day I come to work, my problems are immediately put into perspective. When someone shares with you, 'I was just told I only have six months to live,' everything else seems to fall away. In that moment, I simply try to hold space for the gravity of what is being felt. I give a hug as tears are shed. And in that moment, we are truly one."

CPSIA information can be obtained
at www.ICGtesting.com
Printed in the USA
BVHW030555120220
572151BV00001B/68